MW01296855

Connecting
the
Dots

The Impact of Sin on Our Health

●●●●●●●●●●●●●●●●●●●●●●●

Lindsay Egli, MA, EdD(c), CHES®

ISBN 978-1-0980-5018-4 (paperback)
ISBN 978-1-0980-5019-1 (digital)

Copyright © 2020 by Lindsay Egli, MA, EdD(c), CHES®

All rights reserved. No part of this publication may be reproduced, distributed, or transmitted in any form or by any means, including photocopying, recording, or other electronic or mechanical methods without the prior written permission of the publisher. For permission requests, solicit the publisher via the address below.

Christian Faith Publishing, Inc.
832 Park Avenue
Meadville, PA 16335
www.christianfaithpublishing.com

Printed in the United States of America

Contents

Endorsements

Lindsay Egli does a masterful job weaving current health facts, statistics, and biblical truth to connect the dots on the powerful and negative impact of sin in our culture. While anyone could learn and grow from reading this book, young adults can gain the most from her insights. I highly recommend this book and hope you start connecting the dots to a better life in Christ.

Al Robertson
Pastor & Author
Star of A&E's Duck Dynasty

Connecting the Dots skillfully connects two sets of dots in its power-packed pages. By connecting God's revelation in Scripture with His revelation in Creation, Lindsay Egli demonstrates how healthy living aligns with God's design. And by connecting the dots that define what it means to be human, she shows how integrating faith in every aspect of our lives is the key to walking in wellness. In an enjoyable conversational style, this book truly connects the dots for anyone who wants to live their life as God intended. You will benefit from reading this book.

Dondi E. Costin, Ph.D.
Major General, U.S. Air Force, Retired
President, Charleston Southern University

I know Lindsay Egli as a wonderful mother to her children, wife to her husband, and devoted follower of Christ. She is also a first-rate teacher and is faithful in teaching this generation not only the discipline in which she is an expert but also in the truth of the Scriptures. This book is going to resonate with students and connect them with wisdom. The book is full of gems. There are some comments she makes about various topics she addresses that are the best I have read on the topic. I will let the reader mine the book for those truths. I highly recommend Lindsay and her book!

Dr. Gregory V. Hall
President Emeritus
Warner University

I dedicate this book to my husband Brent. Brent is living proof the Spirit can take a life of sin and renew it in His name and for His glory. My husband has always championed and encouraged me to succeed, held me accountable, and challenged me to be a better person. He is the spiritual leader of our home, a fantastic father, and a wonderful husband. Thank you Brent (Eggs) for your witness and your testimony. You inspire me. To God be the glory!

Introduction

I have come to realize in my faith journey that there is a great disconnect today. Christians and non-Christians alike have trouble connecting the dots. We learn cause and effect early on in school, in church, and from the people around us. We learn the idea of consequences as toddlers and yet still struggle with the idea as adults. Why is this? Have you ever noticed we expect good things to happen when we do something right but get "bent out of shape" when we are forced to face the consequences after doing something wrong? Let me tell you a little bit about myself and why I believe the Holy Spirit led me to write this book.

My name is Lindsay Egli. You have likely never heard of me, unless you followed the University of Florida softball team in 2005 and 2006 or are involved in the softball community in central Florida. I grew up in a Christian home. I was raised in church and knew the well-known Bible stories. I could have told you the story of David and the Goliath but could not have told you what happened on the road to Damascus. I was baptized in early elementary school and, most certainly, believed in God, but I did not walk in life-changing, saving faith until the end of my time at the University of Florida. My family was heavily involved in sports, so we spent most weekends of the year traveling around the nation, playing in major fastpitch softball tournaments. I was a pitcher and began to advance and develop in my skills. In high school, my team earned four-state championships, and I went on to play at the University of Florida, until an injury ended my career. Because softball was my idol, and it took all my time and attention, I hit a major crossroad when I stopped playing. What's next? Lindsay Littlejohn (maiden name), the softball player, was over, and now I had to figure out what in the world I was going to do. Within the next year, I came to know Christ on a personal level. He had a lot of work to do with me since I had placed Him second fiddle most of my life. I had to learn to become completely dependent on Him, to die to myself and rely on Him. The next ten years, God was at work in my life. He was teaching me hard lessons and forcing me to rely on the Spirit I now had inside of me. It was a tough time but a valuable time. Those ten years were tough mentally, physically and, at times, spiritually, but I look back on those years, thankful for all the Lord did to show me His strength, love, grace, and mercy. I learned it is not about me but all about Him.

Who am I today? My name is Lindsay Egli. I am an assistant professor of public health at Charleston Southern University in Charleston, South Carolina. I am a wife, mother, daughter, sister, employee, and friend. But most importantly, I am a servant of Christ. God has placed it on my heart to reveal how a life of obedience to His word leads to health, and how a life of disobedience leads to death. I want to take you chapter by chapter, showing you how sinful behaviors always lead to negative health consequences. We are going to use scripture and health education to connect the dots.

Chapter 1

Obedience

I am a health educator. One of the most challenging parts of my job is readily available information. Correction, one of the most challenging parts of my job is readily available misinformation. My eighteen-to twenty-two-year-old students always hold a device in their hands. They can enter whatever they want to know into a Google search engine, and they will inevitably get a large amount of information in return. The challenge happens when they read incorrect information by an unreliable source and believe it to be true. This is tough for a professor. We must teach students things like peer-reviewed, scholarly sources and how to check references. This aids them in making sure the information they are taking in is coming from a reliable source. This is essential for any type of research.

Now let's talk about social media. How many American adults using social media understand how to confirm sources are reliable and take the time to fact check? The amount of unreliable information being considered as truth is higher than ever before in history. Children are now receiving cell phones at younger ages and are using the internet as their basis for knowledge. This can be a dangerous trend. Misinformation greatly impacts every area but especially health. We have major health crises in America today. Obesity, chronic illnesses, illicit drug abuse, mental health issues, sexually transmitted infections, and alcohol are all on the rise. They kill Americans every day, not to mention greatly affect their quality of life. Did you know that God's word is the ultimate vaccine to these health problems? In between the front and back cover of your

Bible lies the great *truths* that prevent a great number of these issues. The problem is most people do not know it, or they know it but still choose not to read and obey these truths.

> Do not forsake wisdom, and she will protect you;
> love her, and she will watch over you.
> The beginning of wisdom is this: Get wisdom.
> Though it cost all you have, get understanding.
> Cherish her, and she will exalt you;
> embrace her, and she will honor you. (Prov. 4:6–8)

Wisdom is important, and biblical wisdom is lacking among professing Christians. The answers lie in God's word. We must cherish it so it will honor us. Preachers and others serving in the churches around the world need to encourage the body of Christ to be in the Word. We need to read daily, memorize scriptures, place them around our homes, teach them to our children, and hold onto them in times of trouble.

Let's talk about cause and effect. If I am a softball player who never studies the game, never practices, or never steps on the field, I will inevitably lose. I will not be of any value to my team, and my coach, most certainly, will not be able to use me as he/she wishes. This is not a team issue; this is a *me* issue. Christians, if you do not open your Bible, habitually attend church, surround yourself with other believers, and apply the biblical truths to your life, you *will* lose. This is not a time problem; this is a *you* problem. We must allow God's word to penetrate every area of our lives. We need to become His vessel so He can use us how He wishes, and we are prepared to do so. Let me ask you a serious question…take as much time as you need to answer. Do you like to lose? No, of course not! Then start practicing and start winning. Dust off the Bible beside your bed and study! Be a vessel for God.

Teach me, LORD, the way of your decrees, that I may follow it to the end. Give me understanding, so that I may keep your law and obey it with all my heart. Direct me in the path of your commands, for there I find delight. Turn my heart toward your statutes and not toward selfish gain. Turn my eyes away from worthless things; preserve my life according to your word. (Psalm 119:33–37)

Obedience to God's word is protection from the enemy. Do you know when you operate heavy machinery or something that can cause you harm, there are instructions by the manufacturer on how to use the product so you are not harmed? Christians, God is your manufacturer, and His Word is the instruction keeping you from harm. Why do we appreciate the instructions about a machine and read them closely, yet rarely look at the protection manual for our lives? Do not let the enemy tempt you, distract you, and maneuver you away from the Sword of the Spirit. Pick up the Sword and go to battle, lead by example to your spouse and children. Study the Bible with others, holding one another accountable. It is time to stand up and commit fully to Christ with all that you have, just like the apostles. We must become disciples of Jesus; it is God's will for every believer.

In the coming chapters, we are going to explore how sins can greatly impact one's health. I want to first discuss genetics. I once spoke to a counselor who told me every family has a genetic predisposition to an illness or disease. This could be heart disease, cancer, autoimmune disorders, diabetes, mental health issues, etc. This is most certainly true. Genetics do play a part in certain illnesses; that is undeniable. But what are we dying from in the United States? The top two killers are:

1. cardiovascular disease, and
2. cancer.

The top two killers are called chronic diseases. The American Heart Association estimates 80 percent of heart diseases and strokes are preventable. The World Health Organization estimates that between 30%–50% of cancers are preventable. Diabetes is one of the fastest growing diseases in the United States, and nine out of ten cases of type 2 diabetes can be prevented by lifestyle changes. Then we have things like drug and alcohol abuse, which greatly increase your risk for heart disease, cancer, overdose, accident, and other causes of premature death. Sexually transmitted infections, mental disorders, and suicide are also on the rise in the United States. We are in a health crisis and looking for answers.

I have spent the last ten years of my life studying health education and prevention textbooks and the Bible. Friend, I am here to tell you, I found the answers. I cannot tell you why each person gets sick.

"For my thoughts are not your thoughts,
neither are your ways my ways,"
declares the LORD.
"As the heavens are higher than the earth,
so are my ways higher than your ways
and my thoughts than your thoughts."
(Isa. 55:8–9)

But what I can tell you with the utmost confidence, people are hurting and suffering because of sin in their lives. Some are aware, and others are not. What if I told you some of these preventable and premature deaths are a consequence of sinful behaviors in our lives? All sinful behaviors lead to negative health consequences. No one is immune to this truth; not me, you, or our children.

There are seven dimensions of wellness: physical, mental, spiritual, social, occupational, environmental, and intellectual (we will discuss these in the next chapter). When sin enters any of these dimensions, it can have a ripple effect and hurt one's health and overall quality of life. We first much establish what we believe so our beliefs can influence our lives.

Below are my beliefs:

- I believe the Bible is the infallible Word of God.
- I believe God sent His Son Jesus to die on the cross and raise on the third day so those that believe in Him can have everlasting life.
- I believe there are people that believe in Him but do not possess life-changing, saving faith.
- I believe there are great deal of Christians that are hurting unnecessarily because they have unresolved sin in their lives.

What I believe should impact every area of my life, there should not be one area untouched by His presence in my life.

God has given me a passion for health education and has placed on my heart a desire to show people how disobedience can have devastating health consequences. We all want to be healthy and for our loved ones to be healthy. We want a good quality of life, and we want to feel joyful and happy. Our lives will inevitably be filled with ups and downs and different seasons for different reasons. There is not a self-help book that can change those facts. But there is a mighty God who will walk with you through all seasons. Place all your trust in Him and allow Him to do a mighty work in you.

> There is a time for everything,
> and a season for every activity under the heavens:
> a time to be born and a time to die,
> a time to plant and a time to uproot,
> a time to kill and a time to heal,
> a time to tear down and a time to build,
> a time to weep and a time to laugh,
> a time to mourn and a time to dance,
> a time to scatter stones and a time to gather them,
> a time to embrace and a time to refrain from embracing,
> a time to search and a time to give up,

a time to keep and a time to throw away,
a time to tear and a time to mend,
a time to be silent and a time to speak,
a time to love and a time to hate,
a time for war and a time for peace. (Eccles. 3:1–8)

This is one of my mom's favorite verses. There is so much truth and beauty in this passage. I am not telling you the content in this book will prevent you from ever being sick or ever hurting; that is not the intent. The intent of this book is to reveal how a lack of obedience will lead to negative and preventable health consequences. The Bible and our health are connected. There are answers to the different health crises we face today in God's Holy Word. Let's explore some of them together.

Chapter 2

Seven Dimensions of Wellness

People often think there are two things you must do in order to be healthy—eat right and exercise. Now these are both excellent things to do for your health; however, these two things alone are not what makes a person healthy. Let's first talk about the difference between health and wellness. Health is speaking more in reference to the absence of disease, and wellness is more about personal lifestyle choices that promote good health. There are seven dimensions of wellness: physical, mental/emotional, spiritual, intellectual, social, occupational, and environmental.

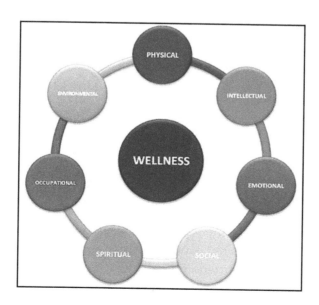

Each of these areas work together to promote health. If a person ignores one of these areas, it could create a ripple effect and lead to illness or disease. Let's go through them together one by one and see what the Bible has to say about these areas.

Physical health—is taking proper care of our body so it can function optimally. This includes exercising, getting enough sleep, eating right, etc. These are all very important areas. We live in a society where many jobs are sedentary, food is fast, and portion sizes are large. Physical activity has declined in the workplace due to the advancements in technology. All of these are contributors to the rise in obesity. When we are consuming more and burning less (energy/calories), weight gain will result. The sins we mostly talk about dealing with food are typically gluttony and idolatry, or you will hear people say they are "addicted to food" (we will talk more about addiction in a later chapter). The negative health effects directly associated with obesity are, but not limited to, the following:

- all causes of death (mortality),
- high blood pressure and cholesterol,
- type 2 diabetes,
- coronary heart disease,
- sleep apnea,
- cancer,
- depression,
- body pain,
- infertility.

We see that not being in control or giving in to temptations with food can have devastating consequences. Physical activity does not have to be highly advanced in order to promote health. The American Heart Association recommends 150 minutes (2.5 hours) of heart pumping physical activity per week. This can be walking, running, vacuuming, dancing, swimming, or any other activity that gets your heart pumping. Doctors across the nation will tell you physical activity is important, but what you eat matters more when it comes to weight loss. The combination of physical activity and good nutrition are the gold standard. As far as nutrition, you first must be in control. If you lack discipline, find it! Control meal portions and eat all six essential nutrients—carbohydrates, fats, proteins, minerals, vitamins, and water. (Your body needs all six, that's why they are called essential.) Don't buy it if you shouldn't eat it. Find someone to hold you accountable. It's not going to be easy to lose weight, but it is necessary to improve your health. God wants to be Lord over every area of your life. Give this one over to Him, while doing your part. Make the hard choices and start forming good habits.

Mental/Emotional health—refers to our emotional and mental state. Our emotions can negatively impact our mental health with feelings of anger, jealousy, doubt, and fear. If left unchecked, these can cause depression, anxiety, and other mental health disorders. It is imperative that Christians understand they can control their own thoughts, guided by the Holy Spirit. The Bible has a lot to say about our thoughts:

> We demolish arguments and every pretension that sets itself up against the knowledge of God, and we take captive every thought to make it obedient to Christ. (2 Cor. 10:5)

> You were taught, with regard to your former way of life, to put off your old self, which is being corrupted by its deceitful desires; to be made new in the attitude of your minds; and to put on the new self, created to be like God in true righteousness and holiness. (Eph. 4:22–24)

> Since, then, you have been raised with Christ, set your hearts on things above, where Christ is, seated at the right hand of God. Set your minds on things above, not on earthly things. (Col. 3:1–2)

If you struggle with depression, anxiety, or any other mental disorder, it feels like you have anything but control over your thoughts. That is the first problem. You are trying to be in control, and you are failing. How do we typically try to control our thoughts? We consume ourselves with those thoughts. We read blogs, articles, and search for others who are struggling just like us. We talk to our friends, coworkers, and families about our mental struggles; it is almost as if we are trying to research and verbalize the thoughts away. This is not the way it works! When you are constantly thinking, researching, and verbalizing your problems, all you are doing is bringing them to the surface. There is a physiological "toll" on your body each time you verbalize your problems. I am not saying there is not a time and place to speak and try to resolve your mental struggles (I would suggest in the office of a counselor or psychologist), but allowing it to consume you day in and day out is not helping. Mental health professionals aid you in redirecting thoughts and changing behaviors. Did you catch that? Redirecting thoughts, not allowing them to consume you. When you are at your wits' end, you do not need a million different perspectives and opinions from the internet, friends, and family. You need a professional, someone who has been trained in behavioral therapy—preferably a Christian counselor. A Christian counselor will understand the role of the Spirit in your life and understand He is the only way to victory. A Christian counselor understands you have an adversary (Satan), and he is attacking your mind. The Spirit inside of you will work to take every thought captive; you must pray for this. Each time I have a worldly thought, I recite Philippians 4:8.

> Finally, brothers and sisters, whatever is true, whatever is noble, whatever is right, whatever is pure, whatever is lovely, whatever is admirable— if anything is excellent or praiseworthy—think about such things. (Phil. 4:8)

We must guard our hearts, placing ourselves in a position to have good thoughts. Stay in the Word, memorize scripture, sing worship songs, and surround ourselves with positive people; the Spirit will take care of the rest.

But the Lord is faithful, and he will strengthen you and protect you from the evil one. (2 Thess. 3:3)

Be strong and courageous. Do not be afraid or terrified because of them, for the LORD your God goes with you; he will never leave you nor forsake you. (Deut. 31:6)

Trust God will fulfill his promises. He might leave you there for a moment to grow closer and depend on Him, but He is there. Stay the course, walk on, and He will break those strongholds of your mind. It might hurt and be difficult, but the victory will be worth it in the end!

I want to talk about medication for a moment. Some Christians believe if you take medication, you are giving up on God. I used to be that Christian. I now think differently. I once saw a counselor who told me every family has a faulty organ (genetically). It could be the heart, brain (also referring to mental disorders), kidneys, etc. She asked me why it is okay for someone with a heart condition to take medication but not a mental disorder? It was a valid point, and one I pondered and prayed over, which brought me to this conclusion. We are not always going to be happy, and certain situations cause certain responses that are normal (sadness, nervousness, etc.). For example, if we experience a loss, it is normal to feel sad and depressed. It is also normal to experience these feelings for an extended period during the healing process. But if we are feeling sad and depressed without a specific cause or it has been chronic your entire life, this could be an indication that there is a chemical imbalance, and medication could be helpful. Like with everything, if medication is recommended to you, it should be by a professional that specializes in that area (counselor/psychologist/psychiatrist—not a general practitioner as this is not their area of expertise). Pray over it and decide. Allow God to speak into your life, and if you feel medication is the best thing, then take it as God's provision. But remember this medication is not a "fix all." You still must put on the armor of God. If and when the medication begins to give relief, give the glory to God for the provision of medication, not glory to the medication itself. Always remember from whom all blessings flow. Take your focus off your problems and put them on God. If you focus on the problem, it will become bigger and bigger, and God will look smaller and smaller. Instead, focus on God more and more and watch how your problem gets smaller and smaller as He gets bigger and bigger. Let Him be the roaring lion devouring your problems. This does not happen by placing an unhealthy amount of focus on the problem but by placing your focus on the Healer and allowing Him to heal you from the inside out. It took me a long time of doing this wrong before God showed me the error in my ways. I still must hold myself accountable, but I am committed to focusing on God and not my problems.

As we look at the remaining dimensions of health (social, intellectual, occupational, spiritual, and environmental), I want you to take a personal inventory in these areas to see if potential change is needed.

Social health—who you surround yourself with and your support system. How do your friends speak, act, and engage? Is there anyone in your life that is causing you to stumble or has the potential to cause you to stumble? If so, we are called to flee from unrighteousness. You must flee! Who are your children surrounding themselves with? Meet and communicate with your child's friends. Make sure your family is putting themselves around the right people. Get to know other believers, attend church, and small groups. Plug in and get involved.

Occupational health—is the personal satisfaction derived from one's work environment. There are twenty-four hours in a day. Let's say you sleep for seven, work for eight, commute for one, take the kids to practice for three, make dinner/eat for one; that only leaves four hours left in the day. We haven't considered exercise, laundry, or homework. What does this mean? It means that you are going to spend much of your awake, adult life at work. Not on a lake, not with your family but at work. It is important you make efforts to maintain a healthy workplace as the ripple effect could impact you physically and mentally. Begin with prayer; make sure you are where God has called you to be. If you feel confident God is calling you elsewhere, keep praying and await His response. He will speak to you through His Word, opportunities, other people, and prayer. If you are working where you believe God has called you, do your best to build good relationships at work, refrain from gossiping, work hard, and do not be lazy. Remember you are on the mission field.

Intellectual health—this type of health typically refers to one's education or level of understanding. Statistically, people who are educated lead healthier lives. This can be due to better jobs (which lead to better benefits/health insurance), more overall knowledge, and less risky jobs. If you have always regretted not going to school, it is never too late. If you don't know if you can afford it, call the financial aid offices of colleges you might be interested in and inquire if you qualify for potential scholarships or grants. Do not forget trade school or learning a skill. Explore your options. Do not live your life full of regret.

Environmental health—refers to the factors in the environment that can affect health, such as unclean water, excess pollution, or exposure to hazardous substances. This can also refer to your immediate surroundings and cover things like mold and occupational hazards. Be mindful of your environment, understand your exposures and surroundings can impact your health.

God created the heavens and the earth. Think about your heaven on earth. For me, it is a mountain lake. Being in the middle of a lake surrounded by mountains, blue waters, and waterfalls pouring into it, this is my special place. I am in awe when I think about what the Lord created. For you, it might be the beach, desert, or river. When we look around and take notice of the creation God has blessed us with, it is amazing. We need to be good stewards of God's creation just as we need to be good stewards with His finances (tithing, helping others in need, etc.).

Spiritual health—is our sense of purpose and meaning in life. This is the most important dimension of health (or it should be as a believer). When you get this one right, the others seem to fall into place by the work of the Spirit. When the Spirit claims the victory, you do not have to worry about backsliding or taking steps backward because the Spirit has no weaknesses, and the Spirit takes no steps backward. How do you get spiritually healthy? First, start praying and reading your Bible. Read your Bible every day. Every. Single. Day. Even if you feel you are not comprehending what you are reading, read it anyway and pray for understanding. There are wonderful study Bibles available to help with understanding. I like to use the Amplified Bible or Christian Standard Bible when I am studying, and the NIV Bible when I am referencing. You cannot, I repeat cannot, be spiritually healthy if you are not in the Word. Start there and hold yourself accountable. Attend church on a weekly basis and get involved. Surround yourself with other believers holding one another accountable. Rid yourself from worldly things, entertainment, speech, etc. Glorify God in all you do. You must actively pursue God every day. This is the beginning to achieving spiritual health.

These are the seven different areas that work together to contribute to one's overall health and well-being. Allow the God who teaches and protects to be the Lord over all these areas of your life. Do your part in becoming a vessel for God. He uses ordinary people to achieve extraordinary things.

Chapter 3

Connecting the Dots

In my preparation to write this book, I spent long amounts of time contemplating the impact sin has on our life, especially our health. I thought a lot about the Seven Dimensions of Wellness and how each area has potential to be greatly impacted by sin. If you are not a believer or have not accepted Jesus Christ as your personal Savior, you are living in darkness.

> The path of the righteous is like the morning sun,
> shining ever brighter till the full light of day.
> But the way of the wicked is like deep darkness;
> they do not know what makes them stumble.
> (Prov. 4:18–19)

As believers in Jesus, we are called to walk in light.

> For you have delivered me from death
> and my feet from stumbling,
> that I may walk before God
> in the light of life. (Ps. 56:13)

In order to walk in the kind of light the psalmist is speaking about, you must accept Jesus as your Lord and Savior and abide in His Spirit. In this chapter, I want to work with Christians to connect the dots between sin and consequence in order to accomplish two things:

1. Flee from sin and resist the temptation of the enemy; be a servant for Christ.
2. Hold one another (Christians) accountable for their actions.

Right now, we live in a society where it is not socially acceptable "to call someone out" for a specific behavior. If you do this, you are referred to as judgmental. As Christians, we are not to judge the unbeliever, but we are to biblically admonish the believer. Look at what John says about the unbelievers:

> We know that we are children of God, and that
> the whole world is under the control of the evil
> one. (1 John 5:19)

As Christians, we cannot expect non-Christians to act like Christians, but we can expect Christians to act like Christians. Non-Christians do not possess the Holy Spirit; therefore, they are not guided by nor convicted by the Spirit; it is not in them. However, proclaiming Christians do possess the Holy Spirit (unless they possess faith but not saving faith, which we will talk about in a later chapter). Christians should believe in the Bible as the infallible Word of God and commit their lives to following its teachings. As a believer, if you see Christians acting outside of the will of God and His teaching, you can lovingly intervene. We see this in the following verses:

> If your brother or sister sins, go and point out
> their fault, just between the two of you. If they
> listen to you, you have won them over. But if they
> will not listen, take one or two others along, so
> that every matter may be established by the testi-
> mony of two or three witnesses. (Matt. 18:15–16)

> Do not entertain an accusation against an
> elder unless it is brought by two or three wit-
> nesses. But those elders who are sinning you are
> to reprove before everyone, so that the others
> may take warning. (1 Tim. 5:19–20)

Both in our personal relationships and in the church, we are encouraged to hold each other accountable and are given instructions on how to do so in a way that is pleasing to God.

Let me give you an example. Let's say you participate in a small group at church. One of the members of the group is using bad language on their social media posts. It is your biblical responsibility to lovingly approach this person, first alone, and then in the company of others (if necessary). This is a biblical action and not a sin. However, if you are at work, and you have a friend who is not a believer in Christ, and they are using bad language on their social media accounts, you are not to approach them. You do not have biblical grounds to do this as the Spirit is not in them, and it would be sin. What you should be trying to do when you recognize sin in an unbeliever is not judge them but pray for them and do all you can to bring them to know Jesus.

Now that we have talked about accountability, let's talk about the connections between sin and our health. The Bible serves to teach and protect us. When we step outside of what God desires (His will for our lives), we are then setting ourselves up for pain and heartache. Think back to Adam and Eve, ground zero for sin entering the world. Eve was tempted by Satan to eat an apple from a tree she was commanded by God not to eat from. She fell into temptation and look what resulted—both her and Adam felt shame immediately due to their nakedness. Illness and death then entered the picture, along with labor pains accompanying the birth of children. The consequences of sin entered immediately and will remain until the day of judgment. A while back, I began writing potential consequences of sinful behaviors in my journal (see below).

- Adultery—broken families
- Overeating/gluttony—poor health

- Gossip—hurts people/relationships
- Premarital sex—sexually transmitted infections and unplanned pregnancy
- Homosexuality—HIV/AIDS
- Living together before marriage—higher divorce rate
- Drunkenness—anger, recklessness, legal, and health issues
- Foul language—a lack of respect
- Pornography—obsessive thoughts
- Disobedient lifestyle—disobedient children
- Pride—being "blinded"
- Uncaring—people will not care about you
- Meanness—short relationships and isolation
- Abortion—relentless guilt
- Marijuana—mental impairment (short and long term)

These were just a few connections I made writing in my journal back in 2018. What I listed does not even begin to cover the potential consequences for these sins, but I believe it is enough to look at the big picture and begin to connect the dots. Now let's look at some of the things God commands in His word and their potential consequences.

- Kindness—others will be kind to you
- Tithe—financial blessings
- Self-control—in control and led by the Spirit
- Goodness—good reputation/witness/respect
- Joy—absence of depression and anxiety
- Give—receive
- Sober—sound mind
- Discipline children—well-behaved children
- Discipline with food—healthier body
- Abstinence—zero percent chance of sexually transmitted disease
- Abstaining from drugs—less premature death
- Not lying—trusting relationships
- Abstaining from pornography—less likely to have an affair

- Read Bible—grow closer to God
- Avoiding strife—lack of conflict

The connection between the goodness and abundance from biblical behaviors is undeniable. Just as the pain, heartache, and negative health consequences that result from a life of disobedience are undeniable. If you love your Christian brothers and sisters and see them stray in an area of their lives, correct them. Think about how much pain you could prevent them by applying the accountability teaching in the New Testament. We teach our children to look both ways before they cross the street, knowing if they do not, it could lead to death. If they do not look both ways, we correct them because we love them and want the best for them. Sometimes, more mature Christians can see things new believers cannot through the discernment of the Spirit. Just like a mother can see the danger of the road her child cannot. It is our job to walk alongside other believers, just as a mother walks alongside her children. If you are approached by a believer about a behavior, I would encourage you to listen and pray about it. Try to avoid getting angry or having an outburst. They just might be saving your life.

Take some time to reread the bulleted consequences. There are fifteen worldly consequences and fifteen biblical consequences. Now ponder the consequences to worldly versus biblical behaviors. Determine how they could potentially impact your health, whether negative or positive. The health consequences that result from disobedient behaviors are devastating. We cannot keep touching a hot oven expecting it is not going to be hot. It is hot, and it will burn you! We must connect the dots, repent, abide in the Spirit, and set ourselves up for a healthy life.

Chapter 4

Addiction

In this chapter, I want to bring our attention to addiction. Addictions can be either chemical or nonchemical. Chemical addiction means that you are addicted to a certain substance, and your body has become dependent on that substance. If you remove the substance, your body will withdraw from its absence. Withdrawal symptoms can range from mild to severe. Let's consider caffeine for a moment. If you are anything like me, the first thing you think about when you wake up in the morning is how fast you can get a cup of coffee. When I was pregnant, I would discontinue drinking caffeine. The first couple of days I stopped drinking coffee were the worst as headaches and fatigue were immediate. See, my body had become dependent on the caffeine. When I stopped consuming caffeinated drinks, my body began to go into withdrawal (in the form of headache and fatigue). Eventually, my body would adjust back to "normal," and the withdrawal symptoms would subside. This same process occurred when I was pregnant with all three of my daughters. Typically, the stronger the drug (caffeine is mild), the worse the withdrawal symptoms. This is what can keep drug users trapped. Withdrawal from stronger drugs might require the help of medical professionals. Examples of chemical addictions are alcohol, prescription pills, marijuana, methamphetamine, cocaine, tobacco, etc. With chemical addiction, addicts are both physically and mentally addicted to the drug.

Nonchemical addictions work differently. There is not a physical dependence; therefore, the addict will not experience physical withdrawals. These are mental addictions. Examples of nonchemical addictions are gambling, sex, food, technology, shopping, etc. These addicts are consumed by thoughts of the addiction, which influence their behaviors. In the United States, more and more people are claiming to suffer from nonchemical addictions.

Now that we understand addiction, as believers, we need to connect the dots between sin and addiction. First, have you ever noticed someone going to a support group because they are addicted to being kind, green beans, or helping others? Of course not; that would be absurd! The reason why is addictions are bad things, right? They destroy families, hurt bodies, and lead to financial ruin. Kindness, green beans, and helping others do not hurt us. Do you see where I am going with this? Do you want to know another word for addiction? Sin. It's not a popular word; it is so unpopular even churches avoid talking about it (although they shouldn't). Do me a favor, open your Bible and find the word addiction. You won't find that word in most translations, but you will find the word sin spoken constantly throughout every translation of the Bible. Look at these scriptures about sin:

> Whoever knows the right thing to do and fails to do it, for him it is sin. (James 4:17)

> But each person is tempted when he is lured and enticed by his own desire. Then desire when it has conceived gives birth to sin, and sin when it is fully grown brings forth death. (James 1:14–15)

To summarize these two scriptures, if you know something is wrong but you do it anyway, it is sin. If you give into your own desires, it will create sin in your life, and the sin in your life will create negative consequences which lead to death. Those that allow sin in their lives will suffer greatly, until it is removed.

Now let's talk about the difference between the world's view and a Christian worldview. The world will tell you that addiction is a disease. As a Christian, if you believe that addiction is a disease, that is like saying sin is a disease. Addiction began with a choice, just like sin. A person has the power to choose to stop an addiction and the power to choose to stop sinning. Let me use Type 1 diabetes as an example. Type 1 diabetes is not a choice; it is a disease. Without divine intervention, a person with Type 1 diabetes will be insulin dependent throughout their entire lives. They cannot choose not to have Type 1 diabetes. They were born with it. We were born in a fallen world, but in Christ, we are not born to fall. Christians, be careful calling addiction a disease because if you call something a disease, you are claiming it is not a choice, and that is incorrect information. Sin is a choice. Eve chose to eat the apple that brought sin into the world, no different than people are choosing to sin each day. If you are going to battle addiction, you must call it what it is—sin.

Now for the good news—Jesus defeated sin on the cross. Even though you have brought negative consequences into your life, if you believe in Jesus and possess saving faith (life-changing faith), His Spirit richly dwells in you. You have the power inside of you to overcome your addiction (the sin in your life). The enemy wants nothing more than for you to believe that you have a disease called addiction, it cannot be helped, and will be something you are stuck with the rest of your life. Do not allow the enemy and the world to tell you this nonsense. This is not biblical thinking. You need to surrender this area of your life to God and allow Him to work mightily and heal you from the inside out. You cannot do this on your own, but you can through Christ Jesus. Do not walk around with a defeated mind-set, stating, "I can't do it." Pick up the Word of God and begin to learn *whose* you are and claim the victory. Christians walk around defeated way too often. It's almost like we would rather be weak and whimper versus recognizing the fact that we have a roaring lion inside of us, who has already defeated death. I would compare this to carrying a $40,000 diamond ring in a plastic bag, instead of a strong durable hard case. Stop carrying the Spirit of the Almighty God in a weak plastic bag, recognize the Spirit inside of you, and become that durable hard case.

> Fear not, for I am with you; be not dismayed, for I am your God; I will strengthen you, I will help you, I will uphold you with my righteous right hand. (Isa. 41:10)

If you are battling addiction (sin) in your life, and you do not know Jesus, it is time to surrender your life to Him. You cannot overcome sin apart from Christ. If you are a professing Christian but continually find yourself entangled with sin, ask yourself if you know Jesus is the Savior, or is He your personal Savior? There is a big difference, and the latter involves a relationship. Believing Jesus is the Savior is not enough; you must repent, die to self, and walk in relationship with Him. That is the difference between faith in Jesus and saving faith in Jesus.

> Whoever says, "I know him," but does not do what He commands is a liar, and the truth is not in that person. (1 John 4:2)

> Enter through the narrow gate. For wide is the gate and broad is the road that leads to destruction, and many enter through it. But small is the gate and narrow the road that leads to life, and only a few find it. (Matt. 7:13–14)

I spent a lot of my life thinking I was saved, when I was not. I believed in Jesus and went to church, but I had not allowed Him to be the Lord of my life. I was lying to myself. When I truly became saved in college and began to let God rule in my life, the Spirit began to change me from inside out. The behaviors in my life that did not align with God's word, were matched with unwavering conviction. The Spirit was sanctifying me and working to make me more like Him. It was not easy; it was very difficult to overcome bad thoughts and behaviors, and I am still a work in progress today (we should always strive to be more like Jesus). I am not saying that if you struggle with sin, you are not saved, that is all Christians. But if you are not feeling the conviction from the Spirit, you need to take a personal inventory of your faith in Jesus. Do you have faith or saving faith in Jesus Christ? I do not want any of my readers to believe they are truly saved if they are not. This is a dead-end road; trust me. The enemy wants you to believe you know Jesus, but do not allow the enemy to speak on your behalf any longer! It is not enough to believe in Him; you must allow Him to be the Lord of your life. Life is precious, and we never know what tomorrow may bring. Seek after God with urgency and allow Him to break the chains sin has over you. If you are suffering from addiction, do not let the world tell you it is a disease. The world does not know your God and what He can do. Claim victory over the sins you are struggling with, in the name of Jesus!

If addictions (sins) are left unchecked, they will cause pain and heartache that will wreak havoc on your life. They can affect your health, relationships, finances, witness, and will, eventually, lead to death. Do not allow sin to rule in your life any longer and walk in peace giving God the glory!

Chapter 5

Alcohol

The debate about alcohol between Christians has been around long before I was born, and it will likely be around long after my life ends. In this chapter, I want to avoid a theological debate and focus more on the health effects that result from drinking, "gray areas," and our witness as Christians.

Let's start with the idea of being sober. The act of being sober is not being drunk. This is often considered when we refer to someone who is sober minded, which refers to someone who is sensible and logical. Do you often associate drinking with sensible and logical speech or action? Probably not. Even though Christians will debate whether drinking is a sin, they most always agree that being drunk is a sin. Let's look at some of the verses in the Bible about drunkenness.

> The acts of the flesh are obvious: sexual immorality, impurity and debauchery; idolatry and witchcraft; hatred, discord, jealousy, fits of rage, selfish ambition, dissensions, factions, envy; <u>drunkenness</u>, orgies, and the like. I warn you, as I did before, that those who live like this will not inherit the kingdom of God. (Gal. 5:19–21, emphasis mine)

> Let us behave decently, as in the daytime, not in
> carousing and <u>drunkenness</u>, not in sexual immoral-
> ity and debauchery, not in dissension and jealousy.
> Rather, clothe yourselves with the Lord Jesus Christ,
> and do not think about how to gratify the desires of
> the flesh. (Rom. 13:13–14, emphasis mine)

The Bible makes it very clear that Christians are not to be drunk. We are to be sensible, of sound mind, and worthy of respect always. This can be challenging even without alcohol, but through His Spirit, we are able. Now let's talk about the "gray area" of drunkenness. By doing this, we need to determine what is an acceptable amount to drink without becoming drunk. I would like to take a secular approach to this thought, with operating a motor vehicle. The legal limit to drink and drive is a BAC (blood alcohol content) of less than 0.08 percent. If you take a breathalyzer and blow above this amount, you receive a DUI charge (driving under the influence). So how much can a person drink before their blood alcohol levels reach this amount? There are certain variables that come into play like sex, weight, underlying health conditions, and how fast the drinks were consumed. But for the sake of keeping it general, typically, one standard drink for women and two standard drinks for men allow a person to maintain a BAC lower than 0.08 percent. Now that we understand this, we must look at the amounts of a standard drink. This is the standard drink chart:

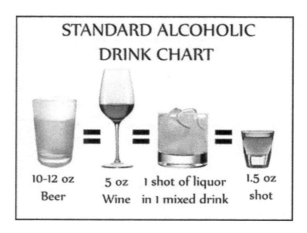

STANDARD ALCOHOLIC
DRINK CHART

| 10-12 oz | 5 oz | 1 shot of liquor | 1.5 oz |
| Beer | Wine | in 1 mixed drink | shot |

Keep these amounts in mind and do me a favor. Go to your kitchen and get out your measuring cup. Pour 5 ounces of water into the measuring cup. It is a surprisingly small amount. Do you think most people who pour a glass of wine only pour five ounces? Probably not, which means although only holding one glass in hand, two drinks can be inside the one glass. If scientists consider this BAC of 0.08 percent to be the cut off for impairment, where do we believe our Almighty God considers impairment (or drunkenness)?

The second item I want to consider is tolerance. What is tolerance? Tolerance is defined as the capacity to endure continued subjection to something. This means the more you drink, the more you will be able to tolerate before "feeling" drunk or impaired. Now we are beginning to dance in a "gray area." If I do not "feel" drunk, then I am not drunk, and I am still okay with God. Even if you do not "feel" drunk, your BAC still classifies you as drunk and impaired. Do you want to spend your nights or weekends in this "gray area" with the Almighty God? I certainly do not. Before I focus on the negative health effects of drinking, let me tell you about my own thought process when it comes to drinking.

I spent my unsaved youth (even though I did believe I was saved) drinking constantly. If there was a party, football game, night out, or boredom at a friend's house, I would be drinking. I was not addicted to alcohol nor did I drink every day, but I was always "down for a good time." When I got saved later in my college career, I began to become convicted and very uncomfortable with the sin in my life. I felt myself withdrawing from some of the activities and friends I had loved so much. The sanctification process was beginning in my life, and the conviction I was feeling was not pleasant. Not to mention many activities revolve around alcohol, and if you do not drink, it can greatly affect your social life. Just ask recovering alcoholics or those who choose not to drink for various reasons. In my experience, alcohol is one of the last things Christians actively in the sanctification process give up, and some never do. It was certainly one of the last things I gave up. It was a process. At first, I stopped any midweek drinking events, then I graduated to drinking on the weekends but not allowing myself to feel drunk. Then when I got married and began having a family, I would drink the occasional glass of wine to help with sleep. But then I came to the realization that I needed to consider every word and action and determine if I was glorifying God. I am commanded to die to self and pick up my cross and follow Him.

> Then Jesus said to his disciples, "Whoever wants to be my disciple must deny themselves and take up their cross and follow me. For whoever wants to save their life will lose it, but whoever loses their life for me will find it. (Matt. 16:24–25)

I had to begin to ask myself if my drinking glorified God, besides, Jesus did turn water into wine, right? But then I pondered if back when Jesus attended that wedding, did they have Coke, tea, lemonade, orange juice, apple juice, coffee, La Croix, and the many other drink options available? The Bible doesn't say. It doesn't give us the amounts people were drinking, the sanitation issues, the fermentation element, or any other factor other than Jesus fulfilled His mother's request by turning water into wine. He performed a major miracle, one we still talk about to this day. But I wonder...did Jesus perform that miracle to begin to show people the Savior of the world had "boots on the ground" or to give people a rationalization to drink? Are we missing the big picture? Are we focusing too much on *what* Jesus turned water into and not the actual miracle itself? What if God turned the water into grape soda? Would we think less about the drink and more about the miracle? After my mind began to ponder these things, my health education mind-set took over. I had already come to the realization in my studies that the words in the Bible serve to *teach* us and *protect* us. When we step outside of what the Bible says, inevitably, it would lead to a negative consequence, specifically, a negative health consequence. Then I began to research more in depth the negative health effects of alcohol. What I found was astonishing.

The short-term effect of alcohol includes poor social judgment, trouble concentrating, dulled perception (especially vision), raised blood pressure, and vomiting. Long-term effects can include diminished gray and white brain matter, trouble learning, liver problems, cancer (throat, mouth, breast, liver, colorectal, and esophageal), high blood pressure, stroke, and irregular heartbeat, just to name a few. Most people believe these health consequences are only relevant to the alcoholic, or the one who is falling down drunk. These are incorrect thoughts and information. The chronic drinker (one who drinks throughout their lifetime) has been linked to serious illnesses involving the liver, digestive system, pancreas, central nervous system, cardiovascular system, bones, and reproductive system. The quality of life can diminish for those that drink regularly. When teaching the death-and-dying section of my wellness course, we are always digging into the life expectancy of different subgroups. One of those subgroups is people who drink alcohol. Did you know most people who live over the age of seventy don't drink? This might be due to a more conservative upbringing, religion, conflicts with medication, wisdom gained from past experiences, etc. Whatever the reason, most elderly people in the United States do not drink or drink on rare occasion in small amounts. What does this say for people who drink on a regular basis? People that choose that lifestyle are often not living past the age of seventy. "Premature deaths from alcohol have lost Americans a combined 2,560,290 years of their lives each year on average. That translates into 1 in 10 potential years lost for every working-age American" (Alcohol.org, 2020). This is astonishing information. People will question these facts, since a study determined drinking a glass of red wine can possess cardiovascular benefits. Dr. Hartz at Washington University in Saint Louis analyzed data and determined that even the lightest daily drinkers have an increased mortality risk. Even with the cardiovascular study, daily drinking increased cancer risk, therefore, increasing mortality. The health effects I have listed thus far have not even considered the problems alcohol can create for a person's mental health, financial health, and relationships.

Alcohol is known as a depressant; this means that it slows down brain functioning and neural activity. Alcohol can and, ultimately, will affect your mental health. Think about a time when you have drunk alcohol. It might have been a stressful week that a few drinks on a Friday night aided to overcome. When you woke up on Saturday, did you feel better, worse, or no different about your situation? Alcohol has a Band-Aid effect. It makes you feel better while you are drinking, but once you are sober, you often feel worse, but now with a headache and lethargy accompanying the original feelings. This is the way alcohol works; it is also a toxin to the body. When your body is exposed to a toxin, it wants it removed. Therefore, people who consume alcohol feel the urge to urinate frequently. It is your body's way of removing the toxin. If you drink in high amounts or at a rapid pace, it can also cause vomiting and diarrhea (also your body's way of removing toxins). In a society where people want all things organic and make great efforts to eliminate toxins from their diets, I wonder if they are considering alcohol as a toxin? Most of us who have drank alcohol can remember a time where drinking caused us to make a poor choice, get into a fight or argument, say something we didn't mean, or have a legal consequence that shadows us throughout our entire lives. Alcohol consumption can have lasting consequences.

Next, I want to spend a little time discussing our witness and the ultimate reason I chose to quit drinking. I had a Sunday school teacher that once told me I was always on the mission field. At home, work, grocery store, no matter where I was, people were watching my actions and listening to the way I spoke. That resonated with me as I had never thought of missions in this way. I began to get convicted about gossiping at work and losing my temper while coaching or in public. I knew I was supposed to do all things for the glory of God.

> So, whether you eat or drink or whatever you do, do it all for the glory of God. Do not cause anyone to stumble, whether Jews, Greeks or the church of God—even as I try to please everyone in every way. For I am not seeking my own good but the good of many, so that they may be saved. (1 Cor. 10:31–33)

I then began to think about others a little more when pondering this verse. First, it is *not* all about me. When you first become saved, you think a lot about yourself. How should I act? What church should I go to? Do I need to remove myself from any situations? The questions start flooding about your own personal journey. As you mature in your faith, you inevitably begin to think about others. How can I approach others about Jesus? Who can I serve? Is there anything in my life that could turn others away from Christ as a professing Christian? This last question really hit me hard, especially about the little amount I was still drinking at the time. I am called to be light in a dark world. Alcohol is abundant in darkness. Do I drink for myself or for the glory of God? When I want peace in my life or a situation, do I turn to a glass of wine or to the power of God's Holy Word? I was convicted. It would have glorified Him if I would have read my Bible and relied fully on Him, but instead, I would have a glass of wine. It kept me from relying on my Savior. I also knew I would face all different kinds of people in my walk with the Lord—those struggling with alcohol, those who were hurt by alcohol, experienced health problems from alcohol, or those that were abused due to alcohol. I did not want to be a part of something that had caused others so much pain and heartache. I did not want my holding a drink to keep people from confiding in me or allow it to be somewhere involving church members and put recovering alcoholics in a tough position. It was for me and not for God, and that was unacceptable. I do not want to have anything in my life that could cause others to stray or turn away from God completely.

I do not see in the Bible where it declares that having a drink is a sin. However, drinking can be a gateway to unforeseen consequences. It might turn someone away from you or, more importantly, away from God. People walking early in their faith might not be able to discern you are having a drink watching a game. They only see another hypocritical Christian getting drunk. Is that fair? Certainly not! But that is the world we live in, and you must ask yourself, is it worth it? Do I drink for myself, or does it glorify God? Could I potentially turn recovering addicts away from my counsel or turn the lost away from Jesus? Do you fear isolation because everyone around you drinks? Do you care more about the approval of others or your mission for God? These are tough questions but necessary in your walk with the Lord.

This can be an uncomfortable topic and often divide the opinions of a church. Myself and my husband choose to abstain from consuming alcohol for our health, our witness, and we feel it distracts us from our mission for God. But some members of our church (both past churches and present) drink, and it is often involved in church member gatherings off campus. We were with another couple who we love and respect, and one of them asked my husband, "Don't you think it would be wise to drink in front of children in a nonsinful manner (not in drunkenness) so we can be an example of how to drink responsibly?" My husband responded by saying, "I can teach my children how to text and drive responsibly (rarely text and drive, always keep the phone where you have a visual of the road, and only text short messages), but is that wise?" I thought it was a profound response.

Christian, is it a sin to drink without getting drunk? No, I do not believe it is. However, keep in mind tolerance, your witness, and the potential health effects that come with a life of drinking. Ask yourself if you drink for yourself or for the glory of God? Make sure if you make the decision, God was included. I can tell you this with the utmost confidence, there are no negative health consequences associated with abstaining from alcohol. Not one. Pray, seek counsel from God, and follow what you believe the Spirit lays on your heart.

Chapter 6

Drug Use

In this chapter, we are going to talk about drug use from a biblical worldview. Before we begin, I want to discuss the gold standard. A gold standard refers to the best or most reliable. As a society, the gold standard for illicit drug use should be zero. The goal should be to promote fully abstaining from drugs that alter the mind and could lead to addiction. However, something strange is beginning to happen in our society. Let me explain.

For the purpose of this chapter, we are going to focus on illicit drugs (illegal drugs). In the United States, our illicit drug use is rising. In 2013, the National Institute on Drug Abuse estimated twenty-five million Americans had used an illicit drug in the past month, and this number continues to rise each year. Marijuana is currently the most widely used illicit drug and is included in these statistics. Now let's go back to the current drug climate in the United States today. Alcohol and marijuana have been the most popular drugs of choice for a long time. The most up and coming "heavy hitter" drugs are prescription pills and methamphetamine. Most people are aware of the current opioid epidemic in the United States, and more people are taking notice of the devastation these drugs can have on a person. Drug overdose deaths have more than tripled since 1990. The chances are high we all know someone who struggles with drugs, died from drugs, or overcame addiction from drugs. You would think with the drug use and overdose deaths increasing, people would begin to become intolerant of drug use. This is where the gold standard comes into play. Instead of Americans recognizing the negative impacts drugs have in the world today and requesting more to be done to prevent drug use, the opposite is happening. We are trying to legalize more drugs. If you haven't guessed, I am referring to marijuana. We have now "settled" into telling our youth the silver standard is best. What is the silver standard? The silver standard is telling ourselves if our children are smoking marijuana, at least, it is not prescription pills, cocaine, or methamphetamine. The silver standard is saying my child will probably do drugs anyway, so I would rather them do something where an overdose is less likely to occur. This is absurd, but it is the reality we are living in today. Do you know how I know this? Because more and more states are trying to legalize marijuana use because the gold standard is "too hard," so settling for the next generation using milder drugs seems best. Or what about when you hear the statement, "Think about how it could improve the economy." Putting money above people always ends in disaster. Let's think about the silver standard for a moment. "It's just marijuana, and marijuana is natural." What if I told you that marijuana can prime the brain (exposure to one stimulus can influence a response to a subsequent stimulus)? This is one of the reasons people addicted to marijuana are three times more likely to become addicted to heroin. Wait…did you just say you can become addicted to marijuana? Absolutely! The THC in marijuana can create a chemical dependency just like any drug, resulting in withdrawal symptoms for regular users.

As a health educator, it is hard for me to wrap my head around why people are against alcohol, opioids, amphetamines but justify the use of marijuana. Not only do we try to justify marijuana use, but we also try to glorify it. I googled "benefits of marijuana use" the other day, and this is what I saw in my results:

- Cures cancer
- Relieves depression
- Improves lung capacity
- Prevents diabetes
- Mends broken bones

Do you know what I felt after reading some of the health benefits of marijuana listed on the internet? Sadness. Let me tell you why. For cancer, the only benefit for cancer patients is the potential to reduce nausea—it does not cure cancer. Depression—marijuana is a depressant with stimulant and hallucinogen properties. This will no more remove your depression than if you were to jump backward six times. Just like alcohol, when you are high, you will feel better, but when you are sober, those feelings will come back. Improves lung capacity—this is the opposite of the truth. Our lungs were not meant to have smoke of any kind in them. When smoke is in the lungs, it reduces lung capacity. Prevents diabetes—not true. Increased appetite of marijuana users can contribute to obesity and diabetes. Mend broken bones—there is not a wolverine effect (*X-Men* reference) in marijuana. If you break a bone, you need to go to the hospital, not to a drug dealer.

This is some of the misinformation our youth are reading and believing as truth. The information is presenting not only a harmless but helpful worldview of marijuana. It is dangerous for youth to view marijuana this way. Let me tell you about some of the negative health consequences for recreational marijuana use:

- Increased risk of cancer (especially testicular cancer in men)
- Impaired cognitive functioning
- Respiratory problems
- Lung damage
- Impaired immune system
- Daily cough and phlegm production

Smoking marijuana can greatly impact your health, both short and long term. There is a definite connection between brain impairment and marijuana, "Marijuana can cause permanent IQ loss of as much as 8 points when people start using it at a young age. These IQ points do not come back, even after quitting marijuana" (SAMHSA, 2019). For something to have the potential to cause so much harm, we have a very distorted view of it in America today.

What does the Bible say about drugs? First, I want to address drunkenness. Most people always associate the reference of drunkenness to alcohol in the Bible. Let's review these two definitions below:

1. Drunkenness—the state of being intoxicated
2. Intoxicated—alcoholic drink or drug causing someone to lose control of their faculties or behavior

After reviewing these two definitions, we can see that scripture is referencing drunkenness as inclusive of both drugs and alcohol. Let's review some of the scriptures below:

> Be alert and of sober mind. Your enemy the devil prowls around like a roaring lion looking for someone to devour. (1 Pet. 5:8)

> Therefore, with minds that are alert and fully sober, set your hope on the grace to be brought to you when Christ Jesus is revealed at His coming. (1 Pet. 1:13)

> So then, let us not be like others, who are asleep, but let us be awake and sober. For those who sleep, sleep at night, and those who get drunk, get drunk at night. But since we belong to the day, let us be sober, putting on faith and love as a breastplate, and the hope of salvation as a helmet. (1 Thess. 5:6–8)

It is made perfectly clear that God wants us to be fully sober. When we recognize that every day we are in a spiritual battle, we begin to recognize the importance of being sober-minded. Think about our American troops. If they were entering a battle that decided the fate of our great nation, would you want the soldiers consuming alcohol, marijuana, opioids, cocaine, or any other drug that altered their state of mind? Of course not! You would want them sober, focused, and ready to take on the enemy. This is the same for God and His children. He knows we cannot defeat the enemy if we are intoxicated; He warns us many times of this in His Holy Word. Will you listen? The enemy wants you intoxicated, distracted, and broken because then, you become his puppet, and he is holding the strings. Is this what you want for your life? Is this what you want for your children's lives?

Each semester, I educate my college students on drugs in America. We thoroughly dig into each classification of drugs and talk about their effects on the body. I spend most of the time talking about marijuana. Let me tell you something about the eighteen- to twenty-two-year-olds today. They know and understand that opioids, cocaine, amphetamines, methamphetamine, hallucinogens, and inhalants are bad for them. Even the ones that are partaking in the drugs throughout their college experience understand it is bad for them. This age group also sees the danger of alcohol and views it as collectively bad. However, there is romanticizing that takes place in their thoughts regarding marijuana. This is not true for all my students. Some do see marijuana as dangerous, but many of them don't. They see it as a natural substance (not enhanced with more THC than naturally grown) and believe it has far more pros than cons associated with its use. I must spend a lot of the time educating students regarding the false information they regard as truth.

In order to stay current on the research of marijuana for medical purposes, my classes spend time studying what types of illnesses marijuana might be able to offer relief. Here are some of the findings (although they lack rigorous testing, like most pharmaceuticals):

- Lack of human study leaves uncertainty in results.
- Still classified as a schedule 1 substance (high risk of abuse and lacks acceptable medical use).
- It contains over one hundred chemical compounds called cannabinoids.
- Since most users are recreational, it is difficult to make observations due to people's lack of willingness to share use and dosage/frequency inconsistencies.

- Potential to aid with chronic pain, glaucoma, seizures, nausea/vomiting due to chemotherapy treatment, or HIV/AIDS transitioning.
- Medical marijuana has ONLY been proven safe for short term use.

To summarize, this is what we know from a health education standpoint. Marijuana lacks extensive trial and human study required by most pharmaceuticals to access risk and benefit. There is research that suggests chronic pain, glaucoma, seizures, and nausea/vomiting (as a result of disease) can be aided by low-dose medical marijuana. We also know that long-term use can result in irreversible cognitive impairment, and short-term use is the only acceptable use. Research suggests even with the legalization of recreational and medical marijuana, most teens and young adults will retrieve marijuana illegally in higher than recommended doses (in order to avoid tax and get a "better" high). There are definite "gaps" in the research, and much is left unknown.

From a spiritual standpoint, we know it is a sin to not be sober (drunk or intoxicated). This can be from any form of drug or alcohol. There is extensive warning in scripture to those who participate in drunkenness. If you are a Christian and are promoting the legalization of any type of drug (as marijuana is most likely the first of this movement), make sure you have not based your stance on the internet but through the lens of the Bible, with much prayer. As I look at our youth today, I see they have a battle before them. The world is now promoting sinful behaviors, from drug use to homosexuality. This will challenge our children in new ways. We must have open lines of communication with them in order to aid them in establishing a biblical worldview. The world is telling our children to partake in things that will hurt them, both short-term and long-term. The world is telling our children to partake in things that will have negative impacts on their health. As Christians, we must begin to connect the dots. We must work with our children to connect the dots. Drugs hurt and kill people. They destroy lives and families, and we romanticize the idea. Drugs cause our children to never reach their potential as the focus is always on the drug, and everything else is secondary. I listed some health effects from marijuana use earlier, but look at some of the health effects from America's most common drugs (painkillers, cocaine, stimulants, etc.):

- Permanent damage to blood vessels of heart and brain
- High blood pressure leading to heart attacks, stroke, and death
- Malnutrition, weight loss
- Sexual problems
- Severe depression
- Organ damage/failure
- Seizures
- Loss of cognitive function
- Overdose
- Death

Christians, this is exactly what the enemy wants. He wants people to be intoxicated and vulnerable. He wants them to suffer physically, mentally, financially, and relationally. He wants them to be isolated and alone, lacking hope. We are in spiritual warfare. Most people start using harder drugs after beginning with the gateway drugs of alcohol and marijuana. We are called to be light in a dark world. Christians, we must stand up against drugs. We cannot settle for the "silver standard" even when the world does. We are not called to lower the bar to the things of this world but to raise the bar to the "gold standard," the standard of Jesus.

Chapter 7

Premarital Sex

Today is tough on our youth. When I was growing up in the 1990s, the exposure was completely different than it is today. I grew up in a time before social media, Netflix, smart phones, and all other technological advances since the '90s. Prime time shows are now filled with sex outside of marriage (with vivid scenes), homosexuality, cursing, drinking, and drug abuse. Not only are these shows on every platform, but the entertainment industry attempts to make the lifestyles look fun and appealing. This can be dangerous for young minds. Especially if they are spending hours upon hours being exposed to this type of entertainment. When our youth spend large amounts of time on their devices, essentially, they begin learning about life from the entertainment industry rather than their parents or God. Let me put this in perspective. If you take your child to church once a week for an hour, but they are spending ten hours a week watching their favorite shows or media, who are they more influenced by? Now let me refocus this idea to adults. Think about the shows you binge watch. Is it full of unwed sexual encounters, perverse speech, cursing, and homosexuality? The answer is most likely yes. If you spend one hour per week reading the Bible and one hour a week in church but twelve hours a week binge watching shows, who are you more influenced by? The Word of God or the entertainment industry? You might say…well, I am an adult, and I am not as easily influenced as a child. This is correct; however, think about the people you are around all time (exposed to constantly). Have you ever noticed you begin to speak like them, using the same words or phrases? We must be careful, Christians. It is ineffective to tell your children not to smoke with a cigarette in your hand, and it is also ineffective to tell your children not to watch promiscuous shows, when you close yourself in your room to do the very thing you are telling them not to do. It is the age-old saying "practice what you preach." If you want your children to say please and thank you, say please and thank you to them when applicable. They learn by example. What kind of "worldly" exposure are you teaching your children is acceptable? If we are not going to conform to the things in this world, we must not expose ourselves and think like those who live in the world. Philippians 4:8 reveals the type of thinking and exposure that glorifies God.

> Finally, brothers and sisters, whatever is true, whatever is noble, whatever is right, whatever is pure, whatever is lovely, whatever is admirable— if anything is excellent or praiseworthy—think about such things. (Phil. 4:8)

Are our families exposing themselves to things that are pure and confirmed by God's word, or are we letting the world pollute our minds? This is important to consider before we begin to talk about sex outside of marriage. Remember the Bible serves to teach us and protect us. If we are not using the Bible as our standard for sex, then we have lost our protection my friends, and health consequences will soon follow. In this chapter, we are focusing on premarital sex (or sex outside of marriage) and the health consequences that can result. This chapter is for you, your children, or your future children. The exposure rate that society deems acceptable to young minds (for sexual content) is unacceptable. We need to be teaching our children what the Bible says about sex and warn them of what can happen to them if they act on sex outside of marriage. It is dangerous, and let me explain why from a health education standpoint.

We are first going to start by discussing sexually transmitted infections. Most sexually transmitted infections are categorized as either viral or bacterial. Viral sexually transmitted infections such as HIV/AIDS, HPV (human papillomavirus, which may cause certain cancers and genital warts), herpes, and hepatitis have no cure. Bacterial infections such as chlamydia, gonorrhea, and syphilis can be cured with antibiotics but can cause irreversible damage to the reproductive organs.

HPV is the most common sexually transmitted infection in the United States. Seventy-nine million Americans are infected with HPV, most being in their late teens and early twenties. HPV has been directly linked to cancers of the cervix, vagina, penis, and throat. Statistically, this is what is most likely to happen to you or your children if sex happens outside of a nonmonogamous relationship. There is a vaccine available, but it does not target all types of HPV. Since the cancers associated with HPV directly involve reproductive organs, it can affect a person's reproductive health and result in infertility or inability to sustain a pregnancy.

HPV is the most common but not the only sexually transmitted infection of concern. When you are sexually active, you are at risk for all sexually transmitted infections and the negative health consequences they will create. The current rise in STIs is a serious public health concern, and many people are unaware of the dangers involved with promiscuous behavior, especially our youth (most people who contract an STI are between the ages of 15–24). Sexually transmitted infections can lead to lifelong consequences and death. This lifestyle of promiscuous behavior is promoted in today's society on many different platforms. I was listening to a sermon by Robby Gallaty a while back, and he made a profound statement. "What one generation allows, the next will accept, and the one after will promote." Christians, I believe we live in a society that promotes sexual promiscuity in all age groups, and the effects will be devastating for this generation and the ones to come. Let me give you some statistics about STIs in the United States:

- One in two sexually active persons will contract an STI by the age of twenty-five.
- Twenty million new STI cases occur each year.
- Undiagnosed STIs cause roughly twenty-four thousand women to become infertile each year.
- STI's annual direct cost is $16 billion.

Do you think our sexually active youth are ready for these consequences? Do you think your teenager or young adult child is ready to get cancer, struggle with infertility, or battle the mental consequences such as depression? I do not believe they are; I also do not believe they are aware of the risks they are taking in participating in premarital sex. We need to educate them. We need to teach our youth about Jesus and His Holy Word. Do you know the percentage of two virgins who have never participated in any sexual activity contracting an STI? Zero. There are no devastating health consequences, no unplanned pregnancies, emotional turmoil, gossip/rumors, depression, or the many other problems a sexual relationship outside of marriage can cause. Not one. So what does the Bible have to say about sex?

> Flee from sexual immorality. All other sins a person commits are outside the body, but whoever sins sexually, sins against their own body. Do you not know that your bodies are temples of the Holy Spirit, who is in you, whom you have received from God? You are not your own; you were bought at a price. Therefore, honor God with your bodies. (1 Cor. 6:18–20)

> But among you there must not be even a hint of sexual immorality, or of any kind of impurity, or of greed, because these are improper for God's holy people. (Eph. 5:3)

> It is God's will that you should be sanctified: that you should avoid sexual immorality; that each of you should learn to control your own body in a way that is holy and honorable, not in passionate lust like the pagans, who do not know God. (1 Thess. 4:3–5)

> Marriage should be honored by all, and the marriage bed kept pure, for God will judge the adulterer and all the sexually immoral. (Heb. 13:4)

It is undeniable that our Holy God forbids sexually immorality. He warns us consistently throughout the Bible to stay away from all sexually immoral acts. We must study the Word of God, and we need to begin to connect the dots that sin can and will affect our health. Once we know and understand, we must apply these *truths* to our lives. What does this mean for you and your family? It means if you are currently partaking in sexually immoral acts, you must stop! Pray to God, asking for forgiveness, strength, and discipline. After you repent, free yourself from condemnation because God's grace is sufficient. If you are worried you have already been exposed to an STI or are suffering mentally from past transgressions, go to the doctor to get tested, see a counselor, and seek counsel from other trusted believers who can hold you accountable in the future. When you allow God to be the Lord over this area of your life, He will not waste this pain. Begin to allow yourself to heal spiritually, mentally, and physically.

> Forget the former things; do not dwell on the past. See, I am doing a new thing! Now it springs up; do you not perceive it? I am making a way in the wilderness and streams in the wasteland. (Isa. 43:18–19)

The next thing I want to focus on is prevention. This comes by communication. We know most of the promiscuous behavior and sexually transmitted infections is among the 15–24 age group. We need to be aware and intentional about educating our youth and young adults. The negative health effects mentally, physically, emotionally, and spiritually can be devastating. Christian, you must be able to talk with your children about sex; if you won't, someone else will. Communicate with them about what the Bible says about the topic. Teach them that every action has a consequence. My whole intention for this book is to aid people in connecting their current health circumstances with potential sin in their life and shed light on some of the detrimental health effects that result from living a sinful life. The gold standard is to educate, which leads to prevention. If you are a young adult, allow God to rule every area of your life. Trust that His ways bring life, and the ways of the world lead to death. Understand you have an adversary that comes to kill, steal, and destroy. Overcome temptations through the Holy Spirit inside of you, who is your sovereign Helper. Do not be afraid to stand alone. Worldly people love worldly company. You are not of the world, so stay out of the world! Guard your heart, mind, and soul from being exposed to things that do not glorify and honor God. I promise you, if you commit to a pure life, you will not be alone. There are others who have committed to being pure; find them. You might need to flee from some "friends" who desire for you to live with them in the world.

In my classes, we talk about sexually transmitted infections and premarital sex extensively. I am blessed with the opportunity to work at a Christian university, and I can implement my faith into our course content. We have excellent discussions during this time. We have "real" discussions. I reveal to them some of my regrets and what I have learned from past experiences. I meet some who are pure and those who are not pure. Many perspectives come into play as my classes contain believers, nonbelievers, and those that are unsure. My mission is not to judge or condemn but talk about the Word of God and warn students about health consequences associated with sex outside of marriage. I urge them to not only listen to me but pick up both their Bibles and their textbook and connect the dots.

I look around, and I see people hurting. I read case studies, view social media, speak to people, and I can see we need light in areas of darkness. I have seen in too many textbooks and read too many case studies where both the young and the old are becoming sick and hurting, mentally and physically, due to engaging in sexual relationships without thinking about the consequences. Christians, we are called to be light in a dark world. We must protect the next generation by biblical teaching and education and refuse to promote these types of behaviors. This will take change. We must take the time to ensure our youth have a biblical foundation in God's design for sex, eliminating the wrong kind of exposure, and being intentional in our efforts to combat this promotion in today's society. We all want to be healthy and must let God's Word penetrate our hearts and guide us to actions that promote health.

Chapter 8

Human Sexuality

If there was one word to describe human sexuality in America today, it should be confusion. Americans are absolutely confused when it comes to determining one's sexuality. People are now allowing their children to choose their sexual identities at an early age. Let's define some key terms before we get started:

- Human sexuality—is the way people experience and express themselves sexually.
- Gender identity—is the personal sense of one's own gender.
- Transgender—people have a gender identity or gender expression that differs from their sex assigned at birth.
- Transsexual—people experience a gender identity that is inconsistent with, or not culturally associated with, their assigned sex and desire to permanently transition to the gender with which they identify, usually seeking medical assistance.

Do these definitions make you uncomfortable and potentially make you want to skip past this chapter altogether? I would ask that you don't. The reason why is you, your children, and your grandchildren are getting bombarded with these terms. They are being taught by the world that you make decisions based on how you feel. If you feel like a woman but were born a man, God must have made a mistake, and live the way you feel. I have a hard truth; God does not make mistakes. He created man because he wants them to be a man, and He created woman because He wants them to be a woman. There is no "gray area" regarding these topics, but the world is trying to create "gray area." Let's think about this flawed logic for a moment. Let's say there is an eight-year-old boy who "identifies" as a girl. He tells his parents he wants to dress and act like a girl because that is how he feels. They decide to allow this; now the boy begins to dress and act like a girl. Now let's say this same boy "feels" like he should only eat cake, "feels" like he should not go to school, and "feels" like he wants to punch kids that make him angry. Do the parents then allow him to only eat cake, drop out of school, and punch anyone that makes him angry? This is the precedence the parents have set. Do you see where I am going with this? What if ten years down the road he "feels" like trying drugs, he "feels" like stealing, or he "feels" like making sexual advances at another person without their consent? Since he was raised with the idea that you can do what you "feel," I wonder what choices he will make? This is a slippery slope my friends, and children today are the *guinea pigs*. We cannot even predict the kind of adults this kind of teaching in our children will produce. The children being in control was never in God's plan. God intended for parents to be in control, raising their children in His name, and disciplining when necessary. Look at some of these scriptures about raising children:

> Start children off on the way they should go, and even when they are old, they will not turn from it. (Prov. 22:6)

> Discipline your children, and they will give you peace; they will bring you the delights you desire. (Prov. 29:17)

> Whoever spares the rod hates their children, but the one who loves their children is careful to discipline them. (Prov. 13:24)

> A rod and a reprimand impart wisdom, but a child left undisciplined disgraces its mother. (Prov. 29:15)

Children, obey your parents in the Lord, for this is right. "Honor your father and mother"—which is the first commandment with a promise—"so that it may go well with you and that you may enjoy long life on the earth." (Eph. 6:1–4)

It is clear the design God laid before parents and children. He wants parents to instruct and discipline their children. He wants them to teach them His ways and bring them up in the way they should go. To raise children any other way is not pleasing to God. We are far enough along in the book to realize when sin is present, health consequences are a result. Let's look at some of the issues these children and/or adults are dealing with, which can directly affect several areas of health and wellness:

- Transgender individuals experience higher rates of mental health issues.
- Nearly half of all transgender individuals suffer from anxiety and depression.
- Forty-one percent of trans men and women have attempted suicide.
- Transgenders deal with stigma, discrimination, and rejection.

These are some hard truths that are recorded from the transgender lifestyle choice. This is also the lifestyle our society is beginning to promote for our youth. Therefore, it is imperative for Christian families to familiarize ourselves with these issues so we can directly combat them with the word of God. If you have children, they will likely have transgendered students in school and will watch shows and media that involve transgender people and relationships. Communication and biblical teaching are necessary in Christian homes throughout America. We cannot depend on anyone else to teach our children; there is too much at stake. Talk with your children and aid them in establishing a biblical worldview. A biblical worldview will serve to protect your children, while sinful, worldly teaching will lead to death.

Now let's talk about homosexuality. Even though the number of American adults who claim to be homosexuals is steadily rising, most people vastly overestimate the percentage of homosexuals living in the United States. Currently, there is approximately 4.5 percent of US adults identifying as gay or homosexual. This number is typically thought to be much higher. As television and media continue to flood our screens with the homosexual lifestyle choice, it will become more socially acceptable, and the numbers will continue to increase.

I want to first go over a lie from the enemy. He wants people who have attraction to the same sex to fall into temptation and believe they were "born this way" in order to keep them trapped there. It is his ultimate plan, and for many, it is working. Remember, we were born in a fallen world, but in Christ, we are not born to fall. Everyone faces temptations, whether it is alcohol, drugs, infidelity, pornography, bad language, or same-sex attraction. We are all tempted by different things. The Bible refers to this temptation in the following scriptures:

> No temptation has overtaken you except what is common to mankind. And God is faithful; he will not let you be tempted beyond what you can bear. But when you are tempted, he will also provide a way out so that you can endure it. (1 Cor. 10:13)

> For we do not have a high priest who is unable to empathize with our weaknesses, but we have one who has been tempted in every way, just as we are—yet he did not sin. Let us then approach God's throne of grace with confidence, so that we may receive mercy and find grace to help us in our time of need. (Heb. 4:15–16)

> On reaching the place, he said to them, "Pray that you will not fall into temptation." (Luke 22:40)

We can see clearly in the Bible; we will face temptation. Just because you are facing repetitive temptation, it does not mean you were born as a captive to that sin. That is exactly what the enemy wants you to believe. Was Jesus born to sin when he was repeatedly tempted by Satan in the wilderness? Of course not. He came to overcome sin. Was Eve created and born to bite the apple? Of course not. She was created to have life and have it abundantly. The temptation we face is not sin. It is the acting on the temptation that becomes sin. If you are being tempted with same-sex attraction, you can overcome it because the One who is in you is greater than the enemy of the world. Jesus defeated sin on the cross; do not walk in defeat. A homosexual lifestyle choice will lead to pain, heartache and, eventually, death. Let's look at some of the health consequences associated with a homosexual lifestyle.

- Gay men are the highest population of people in the United States living with HIV/AIDS.
- High sexually transmitted infection rates.
- Parasitic and intestinal infections.
- Higher levels of promiscuity.
- More likely to suffer from depression or other mental health issues.
- More likely to attempt suicide.

It is undeniable that living a homosexual lifestyle can be hazardous to your health. Christians, we must communicate with our children on what the Bible says about homosexuality.

> We know that the law is good if one uses it properly. We also know that the law is made not for the righteous but for lawbreakers and rebels, the ungodly and sinful, the unholy and irreligious, for those who kill their fathers or mothers, for murderers, for the sexually immoral, for those practicing homosexuality, for slave traders and liars and perjurers—and for whatever else is contrary to the sound doctrine. (1 Tim. 1:8–10)

Or do you not know that wrongdoers will not inherit the kingdom of God? Do not be deceived: Neither the sexually immoral nor idolaters nor adulterers nor men who have sex with men. (1 Cor. 6:9)

For although they knew God, they neither glorified him as God nor gave thanks to him, but their thinking became futile and their foolish hearts were darkened. Although they claimed to be wise, they became fools and exchanged the glory of the immortal God for images made to look like a mortal human being and birds and animals and reptiles.

Therefore, God gave them over in the sinful desires of their hearts to sexual impurity for the degrading of their bodies with one another. They exchanged the truth about God for a lie and worshiped and served created things rather than the Creator—who is forever praised. Amen.

Because of this, God gave them over to shameful lusts. Even their women exchanged natural sexual relations for unnatural ones. In the same way the men also abandoned natural relations with women and were inflamed with lust for one another. Men committed shameful acts with other men and received in themselves the due penalty for their error. (Rom. 1:21–27)

God has made it clear in His Word that He is the highest authority, and a relationship between a man and a woman (in faithful marriage) is the only sexual relationship blessed by God. Any other sexual acts are immoral and a sin against God. In my classes, we speak often about a homosexual lifestyle and the negative health effects associated with it. One thing I have noticed throughout my time in the college classroom is students like to "categorize" sin. For example, my heterosexual students who are sexually active (in or outside of a monogamous relationships) believe their sin is not as bad as a student who participates in a homosexual lifestyle choice. Again, this is not all my students, but I have noticed a trend throughout the years. I must teach and remind the students; the categorization of sin is not biblical. Sexually immoral sin is sin, no matter the type. I have some students who also believe if they live with a girl/boy with the promise of marriage, then it is not as bad of a sin as if they were sleeping with multiple people. I often hear "You have to try the milk before you buy the cow" if I ask why they chose to live with someone before they were married. Our youth are desperate for biblical teaching and clarity. Anytime we step outside of the will of God (premarital sex, homosexuality, promiscuous behaviors, etc.), we are leaving the protection of God's Word, and negative health effects can result. My job as a health educator in a Christian institution is to not only educate students about health and wellness but aid them in connecting the dots in how our lifestyle decisions can greatly impact our health and quality of life.

It is imperative Christian families are having these discussions with their children, providing the next generation with a firm spiritual foundation.

Chapter 9

Wisdom

Now that we have spent some time connecting the dots on how sin can greatly impact one's health in a negative way, let's talk about what's next. Wisdom. Now that we know and understand that our actions can greatly impact our health and quality of life, we must make modifications where necessary. This begins with elimination.

> Therefore, since we are surrounded by such a great cloud of witnesses, let us throw off every-thing that hinders and the sin that so easily entangles. And let us run with perseverance the race marked out for us. (Heb. 12:1)

What is in our lives that does not need to be there? What traits and behaviors are our children witnessing from our words and actions that do not align with God's Word? Likely, there are modifications needed in all our lives, whether it is removing idols, inappropriate television/media, people, etc. It might be that we need to open better lines of communication with our children to create a firm biblical foundation. How do we know what we need to do? Pray, looking for convictions, counsel, and confirmations. We need to allow God to be the Lord over every area of our lives. Things will begin to look different. Your speech, attitudes, and beliefs will start to look different and align more with God's Word. Christians should be different as we are called to be light in a dark world. Light vastly differs from darkness.

Social media accounts are your biggest platform as a Christian. You can represent Christ to large numbers of people with one post. Get on your social media account and scroll back through the last year. What does it consist of? Are you glorifying God in all that you post? If not, you need to adjust the way you use your platform. If your posts are worldly in nature, I would recommend removing them and committing to looking at all your posts through a biblical lens before putting them out for all to see. If you are a professing Christian, you are here for one purpose—to bring others to know Jesus. If what you are doing or saying has the potential to confuse, false teach, or turn others away from Jesus, you need to address it immediately and put it at the feet of Jesus. If you have read this book and are unsure if you possess saving faith, reach out to your local pastor. If you do not attend church, there is a pastor by the name of Francis Chan, who has great podcasts about this topic. I would encourage you to listen.

I felt the Spirit moving me to write this book. I am sure it will take a while to understand why, but I would like to think (from this current vantage point) it is because people are hurting, and they don't understand why. Unresolved sin might be the reason. They might be saying things like I had a bad childhood or bad genetics. Well, maybe so, but a sinful life will only exacerbate these issues. This is where wisdom comes into place.

Let's say you see where many of your family members have been addicted to drugs and alcohol. Researchers believe genetics can influence addiction, so you must flee from these things. Avoid them and avoid the turmoil that can result from consuming them. If you have parents and grandparents who struggled with obesity and diabetes, you must flee from overeating and bad food choices. We need to heed warning from our families as genetic predispositions are real. People that know and walk with Jesus should look radically different from those who do not know Jesus. If your lady's nights and guy's nights revolve around alcohol, bad language, and perverse speech, how do you look different from the unbeliever? David Platt wrote a book called *Radical*. He talks about taking radical stances for Jesus. This is exactly what Paul, Peter, John, and Timothy did in the Bible. The apostles and disciples took radical stances for Jesus, and we are called to do the same. Disagreement does not equal hate. We can disagree with the things of this world without being consumed by hate. Remember the saying "Hate the sin, not the sinner"? This is still true today. We cannot bring people to know Jesus with hate in our hearts. We must love others, build relationships with them, and tell them about Jesus. This is how you bring people to Jesus, and God handles the rest.

Christians, we must spend time reading God's Word daily. We need to seek the wisdom and discernment of the Spirit.

> Let the message of Christ dwell among you richly as you teach and admonish one another with all wisdom through psalms, hymns, and songs from the Spirit, singing to God with gratitude in your hearts. (Col. 3:16)

We must understand and pass this understanding onto our children. The Bible is meant to not only teach us but protect us. Who does not want to be protected? This truth about protection might be what begins to get your children interested in the teachings of God, and it could be what gets you more interested in the teachings of God. Immerse yourself in God's Word, pray, and seek understanding. Allow your faith to grow and mature in Christ Jesus. God wants nothing more than for us to walk in relationship with Him, being physically, mentally, and spiritually healthy.

> Dear friend, I pray that you may enjoy good health and that all may go well with you, even as your soul is getting along well. (3 John 1:2)

End Notes for Christian Families

Health educators understand the value of educating youth and young adults as knowledge received early in life can establish healthy behavior patterns that will carry into adulthood. With this thought in mind, our Christian children, youth, and young adults need to understand the impact sin will have on their health.

Learning this information early in life can aid them in establishing a firm spiritual foundation, which will set them up to be healthy adults. It is time for a parenting revival for Christian families. We cannot allow this world to pollute the minds of our children any longer. Parents must lead by example, raising up healthy vessels to be servants for the Lord. Let's go all in for Christ. Will you join me?

Dear Lord,

Thank you for your never-ending grace. Thank you for your Word and the power that lie within the front and back covers. May we use it as mighty weapon as we battle each day. I pray over Christian families, Lord, that we will not allow the world to pollute our minds or the minds of our children any longer. I pray for a parenting revival committing to love You and walking in obedience to Your Word. I pray that you enable and equip Christian parents to raise a new generation of believers through our own example of living an obedient life. I pray for healthy families who are willing to go all in for You and make a difference in the lives of those around us, being light in a world full of darkness. I pray this in Jesus's name, the name above all names, amen.

References

Addiction Center. 2019. "Statistics on Addiction in America." *Addiction Statistics.* https://www.addictioncenter.com/addiction/addiction-statistics/.

Alcohol.org. 2020. "Effects of Alcohol. An American Addiction Centers Resource." https://www.alcohol.org/effects/.

Alcohol.org. 2020. "Lives Lost to Alcohol. An American Addiction Centers Resource." https://www.alcohol.org/guides/lives-lost-to-alcohol/.

American Heart Association. 2018. "CDC Prevention Programs." https://www.heart.org/en/get-involved/advocate/federal-priorities/cdc-prevention-programs.

American Sexual Health Association. 2020. "Statistics. ASHA." http://www.ashasexualhealth.org/stdsstis/statistics/.

Centers for Disease Control and Prevention. 2020. "Genital HPV Infection—Fact Sheet." https://www.cdc.gov/std/hpv/stdfact-hpv.htm.

———. 2020. "The Health Effects of Overweight and Obesity." *Healthy Weight* https://www.cdc.gov/healthyweight/effects/index.html.

Dryden-Wustl, J. 2018. "Even Drinking a Little Each Day Can Increase Your Risk of Early Death." *Futurity.* https://www.futurity.org/alcohol-light-drinking-death-risk-1882302/.

Dupont, R. 2016. "Marijuana Has Proven to Be a Gateway Drug." *The New York Times.* https://www.nytimes.com/roomfordebate/2016/04/26/is-marijuana-a-gateway-drug/marijuana-has-proven-to-be-a-gateway-drug.

Facts About Youth. (n.d.). "Health Risks of the Homosexual Lifestyle. Informing About the Sexual Development of Youth." http://factsaboutyouth.com/posts/health-risks-of-the-homosexual-lifestyle/.

Grand Force Air Base. (n.d.). "Standard Alcoholic Drink Chart. Official United States Air Force." https://www.grandforks.af.mil/News/Art/igphoto/2000859667/.

Harvard Medical School. 2017. "Medical Marijuana: Know the Facts." Harvard Health Publishing. https://www.health.harvard.edu/staying-healthy/medical-marijuana-know-the-facts.

Harvard University. 2020. "Simple Steps to Preventing Diabetes." School of Public Health. https://www.hsph.harvard.edu/nutritionsource/disease-prevention/diabetes-prevention/preventing-diabetes-full-story/.

HHS.gov. 2020. "Sexually Transmitted Infections (STIs)." U.S. Department of Health & Human Services. https://www.hhs.gov/programs/topic-sites/sexually-transmitted-infections/index.html.

National Institute of Drug Abuse. 2015. "Nationwide Trends." NIH. https://www.drugabuse.gov/publications/drugfacts/nationwide-trends.

Town of Davidson. 2020. "Seven Dimensions of Wellness." Parks and Recreation. http://townofdavidson.org/846/Seven-Dimensions-of-Wellness.

SAMHSA. 2019. "Know the Risks of Marijuana." U.S. Department of Health and Human Services. https://www.samhsa.gov/marijuana.

Schreiber, K. 2016. "Why Transgender People Experience More Mental Health Issues." *Psychology Today*. https://www.psychologytoday.com/us/blog/the-truth-about-exercise-addiction/201612/why-transgender-people-experience-more-mental-health.

World Health Organization. 2020. "Cancer Prevention." *Prevention*. https://www.who.int/cancer/prevention/en/

About the Author

Lindsay Egli
Assistant Professor of Public Health

CREDENTIALS
Health Education, University of Florida (BS)
Physical Education, University of South Florida (MA)
Health Professions, doctoral candidate, A.T. Still University (EdD)
Certified Health Education Specialist (CHES)

Mrs. Egli attended the University of Florida for her undergrad, where she received a bachelor of science in health education and behavior. During her time at the University of Florida, she played softball on the Florida Gators Softball Team. Throughout her time playing for the Florida Gators, she became the first freshman in the school's history to pitch a no-hitter. She graduated cum laude and was on the SEC honor roll each year.

After graduation, Mrs. Egli attended the University of South Florida, where she received her master of arts in health and physical education. Mrs. Egli is a certified health education specialist (CHES) and is currently a candidate EdD(c) for her degree as doctor of education in health professions from A.T. Still University.

Mrs. Egli began working for Warner University in Lake Wales, Florida, in 2010. She was the head softball coach and adjunct instructor for three years. In 2013, Mrs. Egli began teaching full time in the exercise and sport studies department. She was promoted to assistant professor in 2017. Mrs. Egli is now working at Charleston Southern University as assistant professor of public health.

Mrs. Egli's areas of interest are preventative health and linking sinful behaviors to negative health consequences. She is working on including both areas of interest into her dissertation.

Mrs. Egli is married to Brent Egli and has three daughters—Gemma, Emmylou, and Maggie. Her family relocated from central Florida to the Charleston area in the summer of 2019. She is a devout Christian and is looking forward to developing ministry opportunities, promoting health through a biblical worldview.